The Probiotic Revolution: An Informative Guide On The Benefits Of Probiotics And How To Get Started Using Them

All rights Reserved. No part of this publication or the information in it may be quoted from or reproduced in any form by means such as printing, scanning, photocopying or otherwise without prior written permission of the copyright holder.

Disclaimer and Terms of Use: Effort has been made to ensure that the information in this book is accurate and complete, however, the author and the publisher do not warrant the accuracy of the information, text and graphics contained within the book due to the rapidly changing nature of science, research, known and unknown facts and internet. The Author and the publisher do not hold any responsibility for errors, omissions or contrary interpretation of the subject matter herein. This book is presented solely for motivational and informational purposes only.

Table of Contents

Introduction 4

Types Of Probiotics 5

Benefits Of Probiotics 6

    Probiotics Help In Curing Constipation 6

    Probiotics Help In Improving The Immunity System 13

    Probiotics Treatment Helps In Curing Ulcerative Colitis 14

    Probiotics Help In Curing Irritable Bowel Syndrome 18

How Does Probiotics Help In Curing Various Symptoms? 19

How To Get Started With Probiotics 24

Introduction

Probiotics are micro-organisms found in certain food items and supplements. Studies have proved that probiotics have several health benefits. However, this fact has not been officially verified by scientists. Therefore, probiotics are still under research. The two major varieties of microbes that are processed for building probiotics are LAB or Lactic acid bacteria and bifidobacteria. Apart from these two, bacilli and yeasts are also used.

Probiotics are found in fermented food items like soy yogurt and yogurt. These foods are fermented by adding live cultures of bacteria. Studies are conducted to verify whether probiotics have any influence on conditions like diarrhea, intestinal inflammation, allergies and infections. Although the studies are not conclusive in nature, several group of researchers believe that probiotics can aid in digestion and absorption of food.

Consumption of antibiotics leads to destruction of bacteria. It is believed that antibiotics also kill useful probiotics in a person's body. This leads to several disorders like indigestion, acidity and so on.

Types Of Probiotics

Our body acts as a host for around 400 species of bacteria. These include both useful and harmful bacteria. The useful ones are known as probiotics. Lactobacillus, Bifidus and acidophilus are the most commonly found probiotics with our body. These probiotics carry out various useful activities within our body. And one of their major functions is to curb the growth and spread of harmful bacteria. Studies have proved that probiotics help in killing bacteria like candida albicans and fungi.

Lack of enough probiotics can lead to growth and spread of harmful bacteria. Harmful bacteria absorb the nutrients from the food and utilize this energy to multiple in large numbers. The presence of harmful bacteria in larger numbers can lead to various types of toxicity. This can result in various diseases and disorders.

Benefits Of Probiotics

Probiotics are believed to offer several benefits. Majority of the benefits are related to digestive tract. However, they are also believed to help in reducing food cravings. This helps obese people in controlling their food habits. Probiotics are also believed to reduce bad breath. Nonetheless, their benefits consist of a long list. However, some of the most important benefits include their ability to treat certain chronic conditions. Read on for more details.

Probiotics Help In Curing Constipation

- Constipation is a common problem encountered by several people. For some people it is a chronic issue that causes lot of discomfort. There could be several reasons for constipation. Irregular and unhealthy diet is one of the major reasons. Secondly, lack of activity and sedentary lifestyle can cause constipation. Irritable bowel syndrome is yet another disorder that causes constipation. However, just as there are several reasons for constipation, there are several remedies too.

- Before trying probiotics, it is important to know the real cause of constipation. The best way to know this is to try different types of remedies. To begin with, you should try and change your diet patterns. Avoid food items that are too dry. Consume more fruits and vegetables. Include food items that contain dietary fiber. Some of the foods that contain lots of fiber are split peas, black beans, lentils, lima beans, peas, artichokes, broccoli, raspberries, Brussels sprouts, blackberries, pears, avocados, bran flakes, oatmeal, pearled barley and jackfruit. Include all these items in your diet.

- High fiber food can surely help in curing constipation. However, the level of relief it can offer is not certain. If the real cause of constipation is something else, then consuming a high fiber diet may not help much.

- After trying high fiber foods, you should start with a habit of drinking lots of water. Water is a natural solvent that helps in hydrating the bowels. You should drink around 10 to 12 glasses of water every day. Consuming warm water in the morning would be more helpful.

- Next, you should adopt some changes in your lifestyle. Practice some exercises and yoga. These steps should bring some changes and if you are still not getting the desired effect then certainly the reason is something else.

- This is the right time to try probiotics. Probiotics are microorganisms that are found in certain food products. The role of these microorganisms was unknown for several years. However, recent studies have proved that these living organisms help in easing digestion. Our gut consists of different types of yeast and bacteria. These bacteria do not cause any harm. On the contrary, they help in digestion. They also help in proper absorption of fibers. These bacteria or beneficial microorganisms are known as probiotics. Several studies have proved that the right amount of probiotics can help in relieving constipation.

- If you have tried and tested all the remedies and still you cannot find a solution for your constipation, then lack of enough probiotics may be the reason. These probiotics are microorganisms that are not only harmless but also beneficial for their host. You can get probiotics by consuming different types of cultured foods, probiotic supplements and fermented drinks.

- You can also get probiotics by consuming certain probiotic-fortified foods. These probiotics act on dietary fibers, and in the process they produce certain substances that are used by our intestine to promote digestion. While reacting with different types of fibers probiotics release certain amount of energy which is utilized by the intestines to carry out their functions.

- It may be difficult to comprehend these facts. But you should know that these facts are supported with several evidences. Scientific studies have proved that the amount of bacteria present in a healthy individual's intestine is more than that of an individual who suffers from constipation. When useful bacteria are reduced, it leads to increase in harmful bacteria. This can lead to several disorders and dysfunctions. This bacterial imbalance is termed as dysbiosis.

- Dysbiosis or bacterial imbalance can lead to temporary or chronic constipation. If the proportion of harmful bacteria is more than the beneficial bacteria, it can lead to such disorders. In such cases, the harmful bacteria become more potent in causing various kinds of trouble. They dominate the minority beneficial bacteria and render their functions ineffective. Hence, it is vital to improve the proportion of probiotics or beneficial bacteria and yeast.

- Probiotics helps in proper functioning of our intestines. They help in keeping the intestines clean and free from harmful substances. Probiotics also aid in removing the toxic waste deposits from our large intestine. They also curb the activities of microbes that cause inflammation. Thus they protect the intestines from inflammation and irritation.

- Our intestine contracts and expands automatically to produce slight movements. These movements are known as peristalsis. These movements help the intestine in pushing the food particles ahead. Lack of proper peristalsis can cause constipation. High pH level in the intestines reduces the ability of the muscles to contract and expand. This in turn reduces the intensity of peristalsis. However, there are certain probiotics that release acids that aid in lowering the pH level. This naturally allows the intestines in maintaining their peristalsis. Thus, the presence of enough probiotics can help the intestines in avoiding constipation.

- During the process of digestion, the intestine absorbs the nutrients and water contents from the food. As the food reaches the colon, all the nutrients would have gone and only the waste particles would be remaining. However, if there is an imbalance in water absorption it can lead to irregular bowel movements. If the intestine absorbs too much of water, the waste particles become too dry. This would lead to constipation. However, probiotics can help the intestine in balancing its water and electrolytes absorption. This prevents the occurrence of constipation.

- The walls of the intestine produce certain mucosal discharge. This mucus increases the mobility of the stools. Lack of enough mucus secretion can cause constipation. However, probiotics can promote more mucous secretion and prevent the risk of constipation.

- To conclude, we can claim that, in the absence of any other cause, constipation may be a direct result of low levels of probiotics. Taking foods that contain more probiotics and yeast may resolve the condition. There are several food supplements that contain probiotics in high quantities. You can resort to any of these remedies. However, if you are suffering from any other health condition or if you are under medication for any other disorder, then it would be prudent to consult your physician before making any diet changes or before starting with any new food supplement.

- There are dieticians and nutrition specialists who offer advice on various diet changes that can act as a remedy for various health disorders. Consulting such dieticians may help you in resolving the issue of deficiency in probiotics.

- Immunity system is a result of a proper balance between useful and harmful bacteria. Friendly or useful bacteria are quite important for maintaining an appropriate level of immune system. The major role of these friendly bacteria is to fight the invading bacteria or virus. This external virus and bacteria try to gain control on our body by multiplying themselves. However, in the presence of a strong immunity, probiotics fight and kill such harmful bacteria and protect the body against infections and viral diseases.

- Probiotics can thus help the body in fighting diseases like infectious diarrhea, inflammatory bowel disease, irritable bowel syndrome, Crohn's disease, ulcerative colitis, periodontal disease, tooth decay, stomach infections, vaginal infections and respiratory infections.

- Our digestive tract is directly connected with our immunity system. Thus the presence of probiotics can indirectly aid in strengthening our immunity system.

- Ulcerative colitis is an inflammatory disease that affects the bowels. Generally, doctors prescribe a list of immunosuppressive drugs to treat this disorder. However, medicines can only control the symptoms but they cannot eradicate the condition fully. Fortunately, probiotics have proved effective in treating this disease. Even doctors and physicians have started prescribing natural probiotics for such diseases.

- Ulcerative colitis primarily affects the digestive tract. It causes inflammation of the colon. This disease is considered as a result of an irregular immune response of our body to certain bacteria present in our intestine. This condition causes symptoms like abdominal pain, diarrhea and intestine bleeding. The patients suffering from this disorder often find it quite hard to deal with these symptoms.

- The usual treatment of ulcerative colitis includes a dose of anti-inflammatory medicines. Primarily, corticosteroids are prescribed by most of the physicians. This results in a temporary remission of symptoms like abdominal pain and diarrhea. Once the remission is achieved, the anti-inflammatory drugs are reduced or withdrawn. In the place of anti-inflammatory drugs, doctors then recommend a course of immunosuppressive medicines. Imuran is the best example of such drugs. Azathioprine is the generic name for this drug. Even though such drugs provide temporary relief, they cannot cure the disorder completely. Besides that, long-term consumption of such drugs causes different types of side effects.

- Studies have proved that the probiotics or the bacteria found in the stomach of ulcerative colitis patients are quite different compared to the ones found in a healthy individual. The fecal microbiota present in these patients is also different from that of the healthy individuals. Transfer of normal probiotics into the gut of ulcerative colitis patients have proved beneficial in reducing their symptoms. These studies have helped the doctors in coming to a conclusion that probiotics can help in treating this chronic disease.

- Studies were also conducted on animals. When abnormal intestinal flora was inducted into the bodies of animals, it resulted in inflammation of their intestines. The condition was resolved by introducing a pack of useful probiotics. This proved the role of probiotics in curing the condition of ulcerative colitis.

- Probiotics are bacteria that bring several positive changes within the body of their host. When probiotics are given externally, these bacteria travel all the way to the intestinal tract. They colonize themselves in the intestine and start working against harmful pathogens. Since ulcerative colitis is related to the colonization of wrong kind of bacteria, it is obvious to consider probiotics as a possible solution.

- Several scientific studies were conducted to learn the extent to which probiotics can be utilized as a potential treatment for ulcerative colitis. Certain species of bacteria like Saccharomyce, Escherichia coli, Lactobacillus reuteri and boulardii were considered effective. Medical food VSL #3 also proved quite effective. VSL #3 consists of 8 different strains.

- It was discovered that the patients who were treated with probiotics had around 45% higher chance of getting a remission. This is around 30% higher compared to other alternatives.

- In the year 2012, same tests were conducted and the probiotics used were a species of L. reuteri. This was the most recent study. This test was conducted on children and the probiotics were induced through an enema. The results were quite positive. The symptoms receded quite significantly, which proved the effectiveness of probiotics in treating the disorder of ulcerative colitis.

- Although, several tests were conducted and most of them proved that probiotics treatment is fairly effective, the Food and Drug Administration department is not yet satisfied with the evidences. For this reason the studies are still under progress. However, pharmaceutical companies and physicians believe that probiotics could become a possible solution for inflammatory diseases like ulcerative colitis.

Probiotics Help In Curing Irritable Bowel Syndrome

Irritable bowel syndrome is a common disorder that causes several symptoms. In the recent times, researches about probiotics have proved that they can help in treating the symptoms of irritable bowel disease. Probiotics or the beneficial bacteria carry out several beneficial tasks. And one of their major tasks is to aid in proper food digestion. In the earlier portion we have already discussed about the role of probiotics in raising immunity. In this section we will be discussing about the role of probiotics in treating irritable bowel disease.

How Does Probiotics Help In Curing Various Symptoms?

- Irritable bowel disease is a chronic problem that can only be controlled by medications. It has been observed that the symptoms of irritable bowel disease tend to intensify after the administration of certain drugs like antibiotics. Antibiotics kill the growth and population of bacteria within our body. They kill harmful as well as useful bacteria. Thus, a lack of healthy probiotics temporarily gives rise to several bowel-related symptoms. Under such circumstances, consuming food items that contain probiotics or food supplements that contain probiotics can prove helpful.

- The role of probiotics in treating various diseases related to digestive tract has been established several times in the past. Probiotics have proved effective in curing diseases like acid reflux, bloating, gas, diarrhea, indigestion, Crohn's disease, colitis and Leaky Gut syndrome.

- For irritable bowel syndrome probiotics are certainly helpful. However, the treatment should be taken in a proper manner. Experts have advised that you can adopt probiotic treatment for irritable bowel syndrome only if you do not have an issue of inflammatory bowels. If you are suffering from inflammatory bowels, do not resort to probiotic treatment.

- If you are taking probiotics for irritable bowel syndrome, you should understand the conditions required for proper functioning of various probiotics. The food containing probiotics should be refrigerated. The low temperature enables the probiotics to function properly. Non-refrigerated probiotics may not prove helpful.

- It is advised that when you are taking probiotics for treating irritable bowel syndrome, you should also take Colostrum. Colostrum is a special kind of milk which is obtained from mammals during the last stages of pregnancy. This milk is extremely rich in antibodies and probiotics that have several benefits. They are also rich in proteins. In the absence of colostrum, the probiotics may not function effectively.

- When you are taking probiotics for treating any condition related to irritable bowel syndrome, make sure that the probiotics are composed of different types of bacterial strains. This would help the body in deriving the benefits of different types of beneficial microbes. It would also help in counteracting the ill effects of different bacteria.

- While taking probiotic supplements or foods, it is essential to make sure that your body is getting enough probiotics. Deficiency in the amount of probiotics can render their function useless. This is due to the presence of harmful bacteria or the wrong species of bacteria. If the proportion of harmful bacteria is higher than that of the probiotics, then there won't be any kind of positive change in your condition. Hence, it is important to administer the right dosage of probiotics. In order to learn about the right dosage, you may consult a dietician or a physician. In most cases, people take low doses and they do not gain any benefit. This makes them believe that probiotics are not effective. However, it is essential to get the opinion of a doctor or a pharmacist before consuming probiotics in larger doses.

- If you are taking any kind of antibiotic, do not start with your probiotics. Wait until you finish with your antibiotic course. Once you finish your course you can immediately begin with your probiotic course.

- It is a well known fact that yogurt is a fermented food that contains lots of useful bacteria or probiotics. However, consuming yogurt may not help with irritable bowel syndrome. Probiotics are of different species and strains. You need a group of probiotics in order to deal with the symptoms of irritable bowel syndrome. However, consuming yogurt is beneficial for your stomach. It also helps in reducing the inflammation of your digestive tract.

- There is a special strain of probiotics which is known as saccharomyces boulardii. This probiotic strain is helpful in treating diarrhea. However, several people associate these probiotics with Candida. This is merely a myth and the fact is that this particular strain helps in fighting Candida. Hence, do not hesitate to try this probiotic strain for your irritable bowel syndrome.

- If you follow all these advices, there is a good chance of getting rid of irritable bowel syndrome forever. However, certain physicians may not approve of such treatment techniques. Hence, there is no point in justifying your beliefs. As long as you gain relief from your symptoms you need not worry about explaining it to others.

- Although probiotics are beneficial for our health, one has to be well aware of the way they should be administered. Probiotics help in resolving a wide range of conditions like irritable bowel syndrome, ulcerative colitis, constipation, indigestion and so on. The kind of probiotics needed for each and every disorder widely varies. Knowing the proper dosage is also necessary. Hence, it is essential to learn all about probiotics before taking them.

- Probiotics can be taken in two different ways. Firstly, they can be taken in the form of foods. Probiotics are found in certain food items like yogurt and fermented foodstuffs. They are also found in certain fruits. Consuming these food items can provide a good supply of probiotics. Secondly, probiotics can be taken in the form of food supplements. They come in powder, tablet or pill form. Taking these pills or tablets on a regular basis can provide a steady supply of probiotics.

- When you are taking probiotics either in the form of food or supplements, you should take them at least half an hour before your lunch or dinner. Do not combine them with your meals. You can also have your probiotics after your lunch or dinner, but you should wait for around 1 hour before having them.

- The most effective probiotics belong to the Lactobacillus species. Thirteen different strains of these bacteria are available in the market. All these strains are effective in curing digestion-related disorders. However, these probiotics work only if they are taken in proper quantities. Lactobacillus is quite safe and it is the same bacteria that you would find in yogurt.

- Some people suffer from severe deficiency of probiotics. They may have several digestion-related symptoms like constipation, stomach pain, bloating, diarrhea and so on. In such cases, they might require a regular supply of probiotics. They may also require probiotics in higher quantities. In such cases, you should opt for probiotics that are available in the form of powder. This powder has to be mixed in water and consumed as a daily drink. Note that, you should buy a good quality product which is manufactured by a reputed pharmaceutical company.

- When you are taking probiotics you may need to make some changes in your food habits. You may consult a dietician in this regard. It would be more beneficial to get a professional advice on the whole idea of taking probiotics. You may also consult your family physician about this. However, certain physicians still do not believe in the effectiveness of probiotics. So they may discourage you from taking such measures. Hence, it is advisable to consult a dietician. Dieticians can also help you in choosing a good product.

- If you are taking medication for any condition, it might be safe to consult your physician before beginning with any kind of probiotic supplement. If your physician doesn't allow, you can either listen to him or opt for a second opinion. If you feel that you are badly in need of probiotics, you may consult a dietician and discuss your problems.

www.ingramcontent.com/pod-product-compliance
Lightning Source LLC
Chambersburg PA
CBHW072014280526
45788CB00005B/2046